POLYCYSTIC OVARIAN SYNDROME

Why Should I Exercise? The One Hour Guide to Everything PCOS and Exercise Includes Beginners Exercise Programme

TABLE OF CONTENTS

INTRODUCTION

PCOS, or polycystic ovarian syndrome, is one of the most common reproductive conditions afflicting millions of women the world over. Left untreated or unmanaged, it can lead to other, more serious long-term health issues. That's why it's important for women to take speedy action to manage PCOS effectively.

One of the best, natural and fun ways to do this is to exercise regularly. You may be wondering how exercise can benefit you or someone you know who has PCOS. To answer that question would mean reading a book on the subject. And that's what you're holding in your hands right now. In this book, you will learn the link between exercise and PCOS and, more importantly, how exercise can positively impact PCOS and lower the risks of other, long-term medical complications arising from this condition. By the end of the book, you'll no longer be asking the question of how regular exercise can help you win the battle over PCOS.

For more of the latest research, information, blog posts and exercise programmes please visit pcosican.com

So, are you ready? If you are, turn the page and let's begin!

Chapter 1

WHAT IS PCOS?

1
WHAT IS PCOS?

PCOS refers to a hormonal condition that's prevalent among women who have already reached reproductive age and are still within reproductive age. Abnormally high androgen (male hormone) levels or unusually long or infrequent menstrual periods are some of the symptoms that women who have it exhibit. Also, the ovaries of women who have PCOS may form several follicles (small groups of fluid) and aren't able to release egg cells on a regular basis.

What causes PCOS? The exact answer isn't very clear. PCOS may also lead to other long-term medical complications like heart disease and type 2 diabetes. The best ways to minimize your risk of long-term complications from PCOS is early diagnosis, treatment, weight loss and regular exercise.

PCOS Symptoms

PCOS symptoms may start to develop during puberty, particularly during the first menstrual period but, at other times, they develop much later in life in response to something like a significant amount of weight gain. Generally speaking, symptoms and signs of PCOS may vary from one woman to another. However, there are distinct signs that you may need to have checked by your doctor for PCOS, which include at least two of the following:

- **Excess Androgen Levels:** When you have excessively high levels of this male hormone, physical signs can appear such as hirsutism (excess body and facial hair), male-pattern baldness, and severe acne.

- **Irregular Menstrual Periods**: Unusually prolonged or infrequent menstrual periods may be considered the most glaring red flag for PCOS. To be more specific, less than 9 menstrual periods annually, very heavy menstrual flows and over 35 days in between menstrual periods are considered to be irregular menstrual periods.

- **Polycystic Ovaries**: Ovaries are enlarged and contain follicles that enclose the eggs. This may keep the ovaries from functioning normally.

If you're severely overweight, these signs and symptoms can be more pronounced or severe.

If you have reasons to be concerned about your menstrual periods, have symptoms of excess androgen levels (like excess facial and body hair, male-pattern baldness, and acne), and difficulty conceiving a child, it's better to err on the side of caution and check with your gynecologist as soon as possible.

Factors That Cause PCOS

As mentioned earlier, the exact causes of PCOS is unknown but what is known are factors that can increase one's risk of it or indirectly lead to or worsen it, such as:

- Abnormally high androgen;

- Overproduction of insulin;

- Genetics; and

- Low-grade inflammation.

Women who have PCOS are at risk of complications like gestational diabetes, pre-eclampsia (pregnancy-induced hypertension), premature birth or miscarriage, non-alcoholic steatohepatitis or severe fatty liver, metabolic syndrome, type-2 or prediabetes, sleep apnea, abnormal bleeding of the uterus, mental disorders (eating, anxiety, and depression), obesity and endometrial cancer.

Exercise and Its Impact on PCOS

One of the best things you can do to manage or treat PCOS is to make several important and positive changes to your lifestyle, which includes eating a healthy diet and regular exercise. Exercising regularly can provide significant benefits that extend beyond the realm of weight loss, which can positively impact your PCOS condition. To be more specific, the following are some of the most important ways regular exercise can help you with your PCOS:

- Improved insulin sensitivity;

- Lower cholesterol levels;

- Increased endorphin levels;

- Much better quality of sleep;

- Better hormone regulation; and

- Weight loss.

Chapter 2

Common Barriers To Exercise And How To Overcome Them

2
COMMON BARRIERS TO EXERCISE AND HOW TO OVERCOME THEM

When you look at it, regular exercise is one of the best and cost-efficient ways to treat or manage PCOS. So why do millions of women with this condition not exercise regularly? Some of the most common reasons for it include:

- Not enough time;

- Injuries or specific physical conditions;

- Fear of getting hurt;

- A tight budget;

- Lack of energy; and

- Boredom.

Fortunately, these barriers aren't impossible to overcome. In fact, with the exception of injuries or specific physical conditions that may truly prevent you from regularly exercising, I'd say these barriers are more like excuses for not exercising regularly. Let's take a look at ways you can overcome these barriers.

The Problem of "Time"

While it's true that we only have limited time in which to do the things we need and want to do in a single day, I believe that there's always time for regular exercise if you're really hell bent on getting it in regularly. Why do I say that?

It's because the concept most women have about regular exercise is often inaccurate. For one, many women believe that regular exercise means working out at the gym, running on a road or on a treadmill, or attending aerobics classes for a minimum of 30 minutes straight. While it's true that these are the ideal ways to exercise and 30 minutes straight is an ideal exercise duration, anything that's different from it isn't automatically disqualified as exercise.

For example, you can walk up and down the flight of stairs at work or school during your lunch break several times for about 5 to 10 minutes straight, which can give you a good cardiovascular workout without having to go out of your way and devoting 30 minutes to 1 hour. Do it every day or every other day and you already get a good form of exercise, especially if you currently live a sedentary lifestyle. If you commute going to and from work, you can decide to get off 1 or 2 stops or stations further from your usual stop so you can brisk walk for 15 to 30 minutes every day. Or instead of taking the elevator to your office's floor, use the stairs instead. There are many ways you can get regular exercise in.

Another way you can get your regular exercise in, if you choose to go for gym workouts or morning runs, is to wake up earlier than your usual time. Believe me when I say that once you get used to doing early morning runs or gym workouts before work or school, you'll look forward to running almost every day because of the energy and mood boost you'll get from doing so.

Boredom

If boredom is such a huge barrier for you compared to others, the simple remedy is to either make your workouts more interesting or fun or choose a form of exercise that you find fun or interesting. In my case, I make my early morning runs un-boring by listening to personal productivity podcasts or audiobooks while I run. Because I'm a personal productivity junkie and the podcasts or audiobooks I listen to are quite lengthy, I don't notice time flying by and I'm able to easily get through my 30-minute morning runs without any feelings of boredom. Not only do I get my exercise, but I get to learn new things that increase my personal productivity too!

Other ways you can make your workouts more interesting include:

- Alternating your workouts, e.g., running on Mondays and Wednesdays and gym work on Tuesdays and Fridays;

- Mix your routine up in the gym;

- Change running, brisk walking, or biking routes every week or every other week; or

- Set personal record goals and do your best to achieve them, e.g., faster running or walking times, or lifting heavier weights.

Lack of Energy

Funny but the impression of regular exercising making a person more tired isn't entirely true. Why? It's because exercising at the right intensity for the right period of time can actually make you feel more energetic! While it's true that you will feel tired in the beginning, you will experience an increasing sense of energy as you continue exercising at the right intensity for the right periods of time.

In particular, doing cardiovascular exercise in the morning can help you have more energy for the rest of the day. Brisk walking, running, stationary biking, or working out on a Stairmaster kind of equipment for 30 minutes in the morning at moderate intensity can give you even more energy throughout the day. Just don't overdo it.

What does it mean to exercise at moderate intensity? When you're exercising, do the talk test, i.e., talk as if you're having a conversation with somebody. If you can talk normally as if you're talking to a friend over coffee, your exercise intensity is too light, i.e., low intensity, which won't give you much by way of energy or weight loss. If you find that you can barely talk because you have to catch your breath, you're overdoing it, i.e., exercising at a high intensity level, which can tire you out even before you start your day. Moderate or mid-intensity is when you can still carry on a normal conversation but with a slight strain in breathing.

Laziness

When you think about it, there are reasons why despite wanting to do something, you end up not doing it out of laziness. Often times, it's not outright laziness but something else like feeling overwhelmed or feeling that a lot of energy and effort is needed to the point that you might not have enough to do more important things like work or help the kids with their homework. If so, the following are some of the ways you can overcome "laziness" when it comes to getting regular exercise in:

- **Take Baby Steps**: If the main reason you really feel too lazy to exercise regularly is because you think it will require too much effort and time from you, why not start small? Often times, people have the "take it or leave it" or "all or nothing" mindset to exercising. The fact is, you can start in between by taking small steps that you can easily take. For example, instead of going for 30-minute morning runs when you've never run in your entire life, start with brisk walking regularly for 30 minutes every morning. Once it has become a habit and something that you can easily do, slightly up the ante by increasing your brisk walking speed until you find yourself running slowly. Eventually, your small increments can accumulate to the point where you can already run for 30 minutes straight every morning.

- **Exercise at Your Optimal Time**: If your schedule permits it, schedule your exercise sessions during that time of the day when you're usually at your peak in terms of physical energy. Exercise experts say that for most people, late afternoon is the time when people feel more energetic to exercise because, by then, their muscles have already warmed up and they've eaten several meals already. By scheduling your exercise time when you're at your physical peak, you'll feel less sluggish and ultimately, less lazy to workout.

- **The 5-Second Rule**: This is a very popular anti-procrastination principle conceptualized and made popular by self-help guru Mel Robbins. The 5-Second Rule says that to overcome procrastination, you should get on your feet and act to do what you need to do within the first 5 seconds when you feel the temptation to procrastinate. Otherwise, your chances of procrastinating become very, very high. So if your alarm goes off earlier than the usual time so you can exercise, and you feel a very strong temptation to hit the snooze button, use the 5-Second Rule by counting backward from 5 to 0 and getting on your feet at "0" so that you don't give procrastination the chance to set you back.

A Tight Budget

Getting regular exercise doesn't need to be expensive! If you prefer strength training exercises, you don't have to spend lots of money on gym memberships or setting up a home gym with fancy equipment. You can do bodyweight exercises (calisthenics), suspension training straps that you can bring anywhere and attach to any sturdy door (TRX suspension training straps, etc.), or use resistance bands. And if you want to run or brisk walk, you really don't need to spend out for top of the line running or walking shoes because you're not a competitive professional athlete! Or if you want to take up biking as a regular form of exercise, you can just buy a regular bicycle instead of those carbon-fiber bikes that professional triathletes or long-distance cyclists use. Believe me, you can get your workouts in for cheap or even free! Heck, even using the stairs instead of the elevator going to work every day can count as regular exercise!

If you need some ideas you can head over to pcosican.com or there is a sample programme at the end of this book

Fear of Getting Hurt

If you go all out on any form of regular exercise from the get go, especially if you're living a sedentary lifestyle or if you haven't exercised in a long while, then your risks of getting injured or burning out can be high. But if you start wisely and with moderation, those risks are low.

What does it mean to start wisely? One way of doing so is by exercising at a low to moderate intensity for a relatively short period of time. If you're a beginner and would like to take up running as a form of exercise for example, you can start by brisk walking for 30 minutes every morning. As you get used to brisk walking for 30 minutes, you can transition to a 1:1 run-walk method for 30 minutes, i.e., alternate 1 minute of walking and 1 minute of running for 30 minutes. When you feel 1 minute of alternate running's too easy already, take another baby step of increasing to a 2:1 run-walk method, i.e., 2 minutes of running alternated with 1 minute of walking, until you get to a 4:1 run-walk protocol and eventually, 30 minutes of straight running. This can take months to accomplish, which shouldn't be a problem because the ultimate goal is to be able to safely build up your running strength and stamina. Use the same principle of taking small steps for any other form of exercise you want to do, e.g., lifting weights, swimming, playing badminton, etc.

Another way you can start on the right foot is by enlisting the services of a professional instructor or coach for your chosen form of exercise if your budget allows. Doing so can save you a lot of time and effort that you'd otherwise spend on a trial-and-error approach. It can save you a lot of pain and unnecessary discomfort too because a professional instructor or coach can teach you the most efficient and safest ways to build up your stamina and strength for your chosen form of exercise.

I will be creating some specific exercise programmes for women living with PCOS in the near future so please add your email to the list after this chapter or visit pcosican.com, this will allow you to get all the information delivered directly to your inbox on how to get your hands on these programmes as they become available. .

Chapter 3

EXERCISE, PCOS, AND MENTAL HEALTH

3
EXERCISE, PCOS, AND MENTAL HEALTH

In Chapter 1, we talked about some of the benefits of exercise when it comes to dealing with PCOS. In this chapter, we'll take a much closer look at one of the major ways that regular exercise can positively impact you and your ability to deal with PCOS: mental health.

Mental Health and PCOS

According to researchers at the Neuroscience and Mental Health Research Institute of Cardiff University, another potential complication or side effect of PCOS on women is a higher risk of developing mental health disorders. And in a study that was published in the Journal of Clinical Endocrinology and Metabolism of the Endocrine Society, researchers discovered that women who suffer from PCOS had a much higher chance of being diagnosed with mental health issues like eating disorders, bipolar disorder, anxiety, and depression.

While studies have established the correlation between PCOS and mental health disorders, these studies are relatively young and have neither uncovered the mechanisms by which hormonal imbalances like PCOS can increase one's chances of suffering from mental health concerns like anxiety and depression nor other possible contributing factors. However, it's enough to know that mental health disorders can make a woman's experience with PCOS much harder and possibly more unbearable.

The Role of Exercise

More than just improving general physical health, regular exercise is also good for mental health. To be more specific, regular exercise can have strong impact on mental health conditions like ADHD, depression, and anxiety, among others and can help a person relieve stress, sleep better, boost overall mood, and have a better memory. Even better, even modest or moderate exercise is enough to reap these benefits. You don't have to be a competitive level athlete to experience great mental health benefits from regular exercise!

On Depression

Regular exercise has been shown in numerous studies to be just as effective as prescription anti-depressants when it comes to treating mild to moderate cases of depression without the nasty side effects. And more than just being able to help overcome depression, regular exercise can help keep depression at bay.

One of the reasons why regular exercise is very helpful in relieving depression is its ability to effect meaningful changes in the brain such as to lower inflammation, encourage neural growth, and new patterns of activity in the brain that help foster feelings of well-being and calm. Also, regular exercise – especially running – helps release endorphins, which is a powerful hormone that is often referred to as the "happy hormone." Finally, regular exercise can provide you with a very good form of distraction that can help you get your mind off whatever it is that's making you feel depressed, which in this context is PCOS.

On Anxiety

Regular exercise can also be considered as a natural and effective way to treat anxiety. It can help you relieve tension and stress, increase your mental and physical energy, and make you feel great via endorphins.

One way that regular exercise can help you relieve anxiety is by helping you release pent up energy. After a good workout, you'll have spent a good amount of pent up energy, which can help you relieve anxiety.

Another way that regular exercise can help you relieve anxiety is by helping you get your mind off that which is making you feel anxious, e.g., your PCOS. In particular, exercises that require you to zone in on what you're doing rather than zone out can be very helpful. These include yoga, tai chi, or strength training exercises (you'll need to focus on proper form), or sports activities like badminton or tennis.

On Stress

When you're stressed, pay attention to how your muscles feel and on your breathing. You'll find that your muscles are tensed, particularly around the shoulders, neck and face. When it comes to breathing, you'll find that your breathing is shallow. When you exercise, you get to help your muscles relax and relieve tension. And because of the mind-muscle connection, relaxed muscles often result in mental relaxation as well. You also get to breathe deeply when you exercise, which can help you slow down your heart rate afterward and consequently, drastically reduce your stressful feelings.

Regular exercise also helps you feel more tired at the end of the day, which is very helpful in terms of getting deep, quality sleep at night. When you're stressed, your sleep is shallow throughout the night, which can make you feel weak and easily agitated the next day. It can become a downward spiral of poor sleep resulting in more stress that leads to even poorer sleep. But when you're tired and sleepy at the end of the day, deep and restful sleep becomes much easier to experience.

Chapter 4

Exercise, PCOS, Insulin Resistance and Fertility

4

Exercise, PCOS, Insulin Resistance and Fertility

One of the serious health complications that can arise from PCOS is chronically high blood sugar, which can lead to diabetes (gestational diabetes, adult onset or type 2 diabetes, or pre-diabetes). And the primary risk factor for chronically high blood sugar is insulin resistance. Even worse is the possibility that your PCOS may be a result of insulin resistance, this despite the fact that symptoms of PCOS manifest prior to symptoms of insulin resistance. This is because of the fact that two of the risk factors for PCOS – metabolic complications and inflammation – involve chronically high levels of insulin in the body. Insulin resistance is characterized by high insulin levels.

It's worth noting that insulin resistance can impact some women in different ways to others, i.e., some women who are insulin resistant develop PCOS while others don't. It's believed that insulin resistance-related obesity can affect both the pituitary gland and the hypothalamus, which in turn can increase levels of androgen in the body. And if you remember our earlier discussion on PCOS risk factors, high levels of androgen in the body is one of them.

More than just PCOS, insulin resistance can also affect your reproductive system by contributing to infertility. This is because as insulin resistance is linked to PCOS, the latter can result in hormonal changes that can mess up the proper implantation of an embryo. Insulin resistance can also contribute to a miscarriage because it can significantly limit the amount of nutritional support embryos get from the mother.

How Exercise Helps Improve Insulin Sensitivity

Another great health benefit of regular exercise as it pertains to PCOS is improved insulin sensitivity or reduced insulin resistance. In fact, regular exercise may be the single biggest factor that can help you make dramatic improvements to your insulin sensitivity. Whether it's aerobic or resistance (strength) exercises, insulin resistance can be dramatically improved with regular exercise. And if you want to optimize this benefit, consider combining aerobic and anaerobic exercise.

Several studies have touted the importance of physical activity and regular exercise in terms of improving a person's insulin sensitivity. In one study of young adult women – between the ages 18 to 35 years old - who were lean but sedentary, aerobic exercise done 3 times a week for 6 months coupled with 6 months of strength or resistance exercise significantly improved the subjects' blood sugar levels.

In another study of middle-aged adults who were both insulin-resistant and sedentary, 30 minutes of brisk walking between 3 to 7 days per week for 6 consecutive months successfully reversed their insulin-resistance. Even better, merely brisk walking for 6 months was enough, i.e., no dietary changes or weight loss was necessary, although a natural effect included some weight loss. And in another study of senior citizen adults aged 70 years old and older, walking at a low to moderate intensity on a small trampoline between 20 to 40 minutes for up to 4 times weekly over a period of 4 months significantly enhanced their cellular glucose uptakes without any visceral fat (around the waistline) loss or increased insulin production in the pancreas.

Regardless of your body weight, age, or current level of fitness, study after study shows that insulin sensitivity can be dramatically improved with regular exercise.

Kinds of Exercises

While the ideal exercise regimen combines both aerobic and resistance training, your current level of fitness will determine the benefits you'll get to enjoy from any specific form of regular exercise. If you're currently living a completely sedentary lifestyle, a brisk walking regimen or a low intensity resistance training program may be enough to improve your insulin sensitivity significantly. If you're already performing regular aerobic exercise, chances are you'll be able to improve your insulin sensitivity by upping up the ante, i.e., increasing your training intensity or adding a weight or resistance training exercise routine. One way you can increase training intensity is by doing interval training, which is a type of training characterized by alternating periods of high intensity and low intensity activity, e.g., 30 seconds of sprinting followed by 1 minute of walking, which is repeated within a 10 to 15 minute training period.

Resistance training – if your current fitness level is already up to par – can be a very effective way to improve insulin sensitivity. In one study of sedentary, Type-2 diabetic people, performing moderate intensity resistance training exercises for up to 6 weeks resulted in an average improvement in insulin sensitivity of around 48%, despite no substantial changes in body mass composition, i.e., body fat to muscle mass ratio. Another study involving type-2 diabetic and unfit men who were made to perform progressive (increasing amount of weights lifted) resistance training regimens for just 2 times every week over a 16-week period, insulin sensitivity was dramatically improved despite consuming 15% more calories over that time frame.

What about women? Studies have shown that for older women who are afflicted with Type-2 diabetes, an aerobic-resistance training combo can lead to much better improvements in insulin sensitivity compared to just an aerobic exercise regimen.

Optimizing Insulin Sensitivity Benefits

Longer-duration and higher intensity exercises can result in improvements in insulin sensitivity for up to 2 days after workouts. Why? It's because in such exercises, muscle glycogen is used up and any new glucose is stored as replenishment of depleted glycogen stores in the muscles. This doesn't require production of insulin as muscle glycogen stores cannot contribute to blood glucose levels and increase glucose levels. Hence, insulin sensitivity's improved.

So, if you want to ensure continuous improvements in your insulin sensitivity, exercise at least every other day and if your schedule can accommodate it, exercise every day. To optimize the insulin sensitivity improving benefit of regular exercise, consider incorporating a couple of higher intensity workouts within the week.

As an example, consider the results of one study of diabetic, older individuals. Even if the subjects were already complying with their daily quota of at least 10,000 steps daily, simply walking faster by an average of 10% for just 30 minutes for just 3 days a week led to significant improvements in both their fitness and control over their diabetes, i.e., insulin sensitivity. To give a clearer idea, a person whose average pace is 90 steps per minute will increase his pace to 99 steps per minute just by upping his pace by 10%.

Chapter 5

PCOS AND WEIGHT LOSS

5
PCOS AND WEIGHT LOSS

One of the biggest challenges for women with PCOS is weight loss, i.e., it's harder to lose weight compared to women who don't have it. In fact, over 50% of PCOS-afflicted women are overweight. And while most health care experts recommend that PCOS-afflicted women lose weight as part of effectively managing or treating PCOS, it's easier said than done.

Why do women with PCOS find it hard to lose weight, even with exercise and proper eating? One reason is that when a woman has PCOS, her body is practically on fat-preservation or storage mode. Why? PCOS impacts the body's ability to secrete and use insulin, i.e., it makes a woman more insulin resistant.

Insulin plays a crucial role in a person's metabolism as it transports glucose from the blood into the cells that need it for energy. With insulin resistance, your pancreas is forced to overload the bloodstream with excessive amounts of insulin, which promotes storage or preservation body fat, mostly visceral fat or fat around the waistline. So, if you find it difficult to lose weight and you have PCOS, chances are high that excess levels of insulin and insulin resistance could be the reasons. Because part of an effective PCOS treatment system involves improving insulin sensitivity via exercise, exercise can help you lose excess body weight in the process.

Another reason why women with PCOS tend to have a much harder time losing excess bodyweight or seems to have an easier time gaining weight is because of a stronger appetite. Aside from causing insulin resistance and switching on the body's fat-storage mode, insulin (especially excess amounts of it) can significantly increase a person's appetite. It's highly possible that the reason why women with PCOS tend to be hungrier than most women is because of very high insulin levels. If not managed or controlled well, this stronger than average hunger can lead to eating much more food than what's needed, which will lead to gaining excess weight.

A very effective way to control insulin levels and significantly reduce food cravings and appetite is by eating smaller, more frequent meals (every 2 to 3 hours) composed of lean protein and complex carbohydrates. This is the diet secret of practically all professional fitness competitors and models.

Women who have PCOS also suffer from impaired appetite-regulating hormones, which is another reason why they tend to be hungrier than women who don't have PCOS. In particular, this kind of impairment can make it harder to feel satiated. In particular, women with PCOS tend to have impaired appetite regulating hormones like leptin, cholecystokinin, and ghrelin. When production of these hormones are impaired, you can expect to feel hungrier most of the time, eat more than what's needed, gain weight, and have a generally hard time losing it.

The last reason why women with PCOS have a much easier time gaining weight and a much harder time losing it is an imbalanced diet. Actually, it's not just women with PCOS who tend to have imbalanced diets, but considering the fact that insulin resistance is a common condition among PCOS-afflicted women and this puts their bodies in fat-storage mode, imbalanced diets can have a stronger impact on body weight compared to women who don't have PCOS.

To give you a better perspective on this, consider a study conducted in 2010 that involved two groups of women with PCOS: one who ate a low glycemic index diet and the other that ate a regular healthy diet that was rich in dietary fiber. Both groups of women consumed the same number of total calories every day with the same macronutrient portions, i.e., 50%, 23%, and 27% of total calories coming from carbohydrates, protein, and dietary fat, respectively. Both groups also consumed 34 grams of dietary fiber daily.

So what was the difference between the two groups of subjects? The type of carbohydrates calories consumed. The group whose carbohydrates were mostly low glycemic index (GI) registered a 300% better insulin sensitivity and menstrual regularity improvements compared to the other group that didn't focus on low GI carbs. What the study suggests is that that for optimal insulin sensitivity improvement and weight loss for PCOS-afflicted women, a low GI diet is key.

Exercise Programme

Circuit One:

Complete three times in a row before moving on to the next circuit

15 Squats

10 Lunges on Each Leg

1 Minute High Knee Marching at a Fast Walking Pace

Circuit Two:

Complete three times in a row before moving on to the next circuit

15 Bicep Curl

15 Upright Row

15 Shoulder Press

30 seconds Dumbbell Punches

Circuit Three:

Complete three times in a row

15 Crunches

20 Bicycle Crunches

1 Minute Step Ups

Conclusion

Thanks for buying this book. I hope that through this book, you were able to learn how you can deal with PCOS through regular exercise. But more than just learning that, I hope that you were also encouraged to take immediate action. After all, knowing is just half the battle – the other half is action or application of knowledge. The sooner you start putting what you learned into action, the higher your chances of winning the battle against PCOS via regular exercise. On the other hand, the longer you put action off, the higher your risks of inaction become, which can make it more likely for you to lose the war with PCOS. The best time to take action is neither yesterday - because it's already gone – nor tomorrow because that'd be too late. The best time to take action is now.

For more of the latest blog posts, information and exercise programmes please visit pcosican.com

And finally, if you liked the book, I would like to ask you to do me a favour and leave a review for the book on Amazon.

Thank you and good luck!